Crisis In

A Shocking View From The Inside

Emily Hanson

Copyright © 2021 Emily Hanson
All rights reserved.
ISBN: 9798711835875

Also by Emily Hanson

Simple Healthy Smoothies for the 5:2 Diet

Satisfying Single Serving Vegan Recipes

For all those who are powerless to speak up
for themselves

All the names in this book have been changed to protect identities

Chapter One

I've just watched a televised political debate about whether relatives should have the right to install a camera in the room of the care home where their relative is living.

Not for the first time, my thoughts drifted back to my own experiences as a temporary resident in not just one, but five such facilities. Today, though, anger rising inside me, I felt a sudden and overwhelmingly strong urge, in fact more of a moral duty, to warn others of the dangers lurking in too many care homes where, almost unbelievably, there are staff who seem simply to lack the capacity to care.

With mounting pressure from families for closer scrutiny of care homes, there is a genuine need for anyone with actual lived experience to speak out about the reality of the crisis in Britain's care homes. Carers, visitors and, wherever possible, those who are living out their lives inside these walls, need to tell the rest of the world what is really going on, so that something can be done to make sure that the kind of daily inhumane treatment being inflicted is brought into the open and stopped.

Before I go any further, I want to sing the praises of the numerous care assistants in this country who do such an excellent job, who care for those who are dependent on them as they would for a member of their own family. They are frequently overworked and grossly underpaid. They are the quiet, unsung heroes in our community who deserve far greater recognition for what they do.

So why don't they speak out when they witness bad practice? Well, if they do they may justifiably fear that they will find themselves out of a job; even if they're not sacked for spilling the beans, their employer might say they're someone with a grudge or come up with some other plausible-sounding excuse to ensure that their credibility as a care worker is ruined.

How come, though, we are not truly aware of what is happening day on day, up and down the country, in care homes that continue to harbour secrets that amount to, at best, thoughtless indifference and worse, unforgivable abuse?

One possible reason is that relatives are terrified to say too much in case it results in further mistreatment of their loved ones. And anyone who has little choice but to stay in a residential facility may understandably be concerned that they will not be believed. Furthermore, any complaint about unkind words, rough handling or downright neglect could be interpreted as a resident's inaccurate perception seen through the warped lens of cognitive decline. Of course, there are also those suffering from some form of dementia who are very confused and who, although desperately unhappy, are utterly unable to comprehend what is actually happening, why they are being mistreated. They are powerless, incapable of defending themselves. Yet again, if a person is in full possession of their mental faculties but is extremely ill, they may be too weak to muster sufficient energy to protest about how they are not being properly looked after.

Any resident in care has an inherent right to have their dignity respected, their needs met and to be approached in a warm, caring, compassionate and respectful manner at all times. Indeed a good question for any person looking after them is 'How would I wish to be treated if this were me?'

After all, generally someone does not happily choose to give up their independence and spend the rest of their days in care. Usually, circumstances dictate the difficult decisions that often have to be made; there is sometimes no other viable option.

Chapter Two

Undeniably, there are some places of excellence where residents' individual requirements are considered, where the atmosphere is welcoming and stimulating. My friend's husband has already spent several years in such a home. Suffering from vascular dementia for ten years, his condition deteriorated to such an extent that it was no longer possible for him to continue being looked after by his devoted wife. Her own health was in jeopardy; Bryan needed round the clock surveillance to ensure his safety. My friend was not in a position to pay for his care so it's not a question of large sums of money being paid to keep him in a place where he's warm, comfortable, happy and stimulated mentally and physically. His wellbeing is the top priority for those who work there.

Every member of staff in that home strives hard to ensure that the environment is safe, caring and secure as well as being comfortable. They are sensitive to the privacy of each individual and adapt to their changing needs. Families are encouraged to visit and warmly welcomed when they do so.

Sadly, however, this ethos is not replicated in every residential setting. An ever-increasing number of horrific cases are coming to light; incidences where human beings who may well have spent a large part of their lives contributing to society are being subjected to unimaginable cruelty now that they are elderly and vulnerable. No-one on this earth deserves this!

On occasion we become aware of wrong doing after someone has died, when it's too late to rectify the problem.

One instance that troubled me greatly was the death, a couple of years ago, of an eighty-three year old man.

Malcolm and Edith were our friendly neighbours. During the seven years that they lived next door we got to know them pretty well. Malcolm was a skilled jewellery maker before retiring to devote his time to charity work, indulge his passion for watercolours and tend his beautifully-kept garden. What Malcolm didn't know about growing fruit and vegetables wasn't worth knowing. Anytime I needed advice about how to grow anything I would ask his advice. And his wife made the most delicious cakes for our shared coffee mornings.

This active couple visited National Trust gardens and flew, annually, to visit their daughter in Australia until Edith fell and broke her hip. The operation to mend it didn't go well and further surgery was needed. Unfortunately, after that she was unable to walk without a Zimmer frame and relied more heavily on Malcolm to help out. When she fell again and was readmitted to hospital, Malcolm became depressed to the extent that I felt it necessary to ring his daughter to let her decide how to get him extra support.

The following day Malcolm was taken to a care home where his wife joined him to recuperate from her recent operation. When I visited them I was encouraged by the fact that they were together and seemingly well cared for.

However, when Edith was sent home with daily help in place, Malcolm was transferred to a different home where I was shocked to see a marked change in him. I found him slitting in one of the high-backed chairs lining the walls of the lounge. Some of the other elderly folks were staring at a television, which was at the far end of the room with the sound turned off. A few folk were muttering to themselves. Malcolm was gazing out of the window opposite. The door to the garden was open as it was a bright sunny afternoon.

I sat down next to Malcolm and tried to engage him in conversation. When I asked him if he he'd done any artwork he shook his head. "They don't have any materials here," he said sadly.

At that moment a care assistant entered the room so I asked if I could have a word. "Malcolm loves painting, he's done some beautiful landscapes," I said. "Would it possible to give him some brushes, paints and paper? I'm sure it would help to cheer him up." She promised that she'd see what she could do.

With a bit of gentle persuasion Malcolm agreed to let me get hold of a wheelchair and take him into the garden. My wheelchair pushing skills leave a lot to be desired and, as I zig-zagged my way out, I was worried that I would run over other residents' feet or tip Malcolm onto the carpet. But finally I managed somehow to manoeuvre the wheelchair into the fresh air.

I t was a well-maintained, secluded, paved area with a variety of colourful shrubs and flowers in a raised central bed. Noticing that Malcolm appeared to perk up and look with interest as we passed close to the plants, I asked his advice about the vegetables I was planning on growing in my garden. To my relief he chatted, as he always had, about the best way to go about it.

When I left him that day, I was hopeful that he would get the art tools he needed and determined to come to take him out again soon.

Later that week his daughter rang to tell me that Malcolm wasn't up to seeing any more visitors since he was too confused as a result of a urinary infection and refusing to eat or drink. When this had happened on previous occasions he had been admitted to hospital to be rehydrated. This time, his daughter told me, staff at the home had said that it had been decided that they would keep him as comfortable as possible but he would not be going into hospital to be put on a drip. His daughter and wife went along with this decision and in a couple of weeks Malcolm was dead. No intervention had taken place.

Chapter Three

Two years after Malcolm's died Edith was moved into a care home. She was terribly unhappy about the decision to sell up her bungalow, to give up the place where she had spent so much of their retirement. However, she was becoming increasingly frail and reluctant to place additional strain on her daughter, whose partner had recently had a heart attack.

Together, she and her daughter visited a number of homes before settling on one that was not too far from her daughter's house, which would make visits easier.

Co-incidentally, it was around this time that my husband, Dennis, and I decided to move up north. But since her daughter had a phone installed in Edith's bedroom, I was able to maintain frequent contact.

I was relieved to hear that, despite missing her independence, Edith was adapting well to her new environment and had made friends with two other residents. When I rang she would regale me with details about the delights served up by the newly-employed French chef. Apparently, his creative meals didn't please the majority who preferred the straightforward, basic fare they were accustomed to. Edith, however, was always game to try any new culinary offering; it gave her something to look forward to each day and she enjoyed the change from her usual basic menu.

She also derived pleasure from her days out with her grandchildren and the occasional mini bus trip to the local fish and chip restaurant. Edith was someone who accepted life as it was. I never heard her complain about anything; she simply made the best of however things happened to be. I admired her attitude to life. She just didn't see the point in wasting energy on anything beyond her control, she told me.

Despite her frailty, Edith remained healthy

over the next eighteen months. She was delighted when we finally managed to get down to visit her.

When we arrived we were directed to the dining room where the tables had been pushed to one side to allow rows of chairs to be placed. Facing them, a soprano was enthusiastically regaling them with songs.

My hope that we could slip in unnoticed to sit next to Edith, who was seated near the door, was short-lived. Having failed to elicit any response to her invitation for residents to sing and dance to her next rendition of songs from 'The Sound of Music', she seized this unexpected opportunity to single us out to help entertain her audience.

When she'd established our names and whom we were visiting, she urged us to come and join her.

Now, quite apart from the fact that my vocal powers are roughly equivalent to someone trying to cut wood with a rusty saw, I have an inherent dread of performing in public. With Dennis protesting politely that he couldn't sing, the singer directed her attention to me. , "Come on up here Emily, I'm sure Edith would love to see you perform."

I glanced at Edith who was now smiling encouragingly. How could I resist pleasing my friend? Squirming inside, I spent the next ten minutes pretending to be part of what was intended to be fun for everyone in the room. Sadly, looking at the faces of most of the residents present, I wasn't convinced that they were finding it enjoyable either.

With my ordeal over, Edith was anxious to take us to her room. It was a small space, little bigger than the average bathroom. Immediately to the right of the door was a bed with the head of it facing the door. Presumably the rationale for this was that anyone checking on its occupant could see them easily. It meant, however, that the person in bed was unable to see out of the window.

Opposite the bed was a wardrobe and at the bottom of the bed a door opened onto an ensuite with scarcely enough space for the shower, toilet and sink. The one saving grace was the armchair, next to a window opposite the ensuite, which looked onto a courtyard, dotted with attractive potted plants. Edith said she spent a lot of the day sitting there.

I wondered what had become of all the photos she had displayed around her bungalow. Only one, a photo of her and Malcolm, on their wedding day sixty-two years ago, stood on the tiny cabinet between the wardrobe and her chair. There was no other surface on which to put anything. And it occurred to me that the cabinet would normally be used as a bedside table except, of course, in this room it would have blocked the door from opening.

In many houses this room would have been called the box room. Despite its size, I found myself pondering how I would best maximize this space if it were up to me. Having emptied the room, I'd paint these clinically white walls in a calming pastel colour, put up matching curtains and have a new carpet fitted. My next move would be to turn the bed around from its current position, so that the moment the curtains were drawn I'd have an unimpeded view out of the window. That wardrobe would have to go and a slimmer, sleeker version put in its place. And I'd definitely update the chair to a more comfortable, less unwieldy model which would allow a longer cabinet with a greater surface area for more photos. All these alterations would also increase the usable wall space, meaning that a few pictures could then be mounted.

It wasn't up to me though, and it seemed that, despite Edith's acceptance of everything she wasn't content with the way thing were.

"When we were shown round I was shown the room next door, which is a much larger one and more modern and I was told that it would be mine once the present occupant vacated it. They didn't say when that would be though and I'm still waiting. It's a nice one so I do hope I'll get it one day." The bit that remained unspoken was that, in all likelihood, for Edith to claim it the present incumbent would have to die!

At teatime we said our goodbyes and headed quickly for the car park. Once in our car I could no longer hold back the tears.

Chapter Four

Early in 2019 when I rang Edith one evening for our regular chat she seemed unusually worried. As we talked it transpired that she'd been told she had dementia. She said she'd been tested by a nurse, so it must be true. She hadn't had any brain scans though.

Knowing, from my son, who's a doctor, the type of questions that are asked to determine this diagnosis, I asked questions like, "Who's the current Prime Minister?" "Can you spell 'world' backwards?" and "What did you have for lunch?" Edith not only answered correctly but added that they were now condemned to jam sandwiches for tea – a popular choice for the majority of the residents but disappointing for her as she always looked forward to the 'fancy dishes' the French cook had served up. Unfortunately, for Edith, there was a new chef.

Having spoken for around twenty minutes I

told Edith that I couldn't see any evidence of mental deterioration, that, although she may sometimes be forgetful as we all are at times, I really thought she'd been wrongly labelled.

Over the next few months I remained alert during our phone conversations to any signs of cognitive impairment but found none.

In July Edith's phone continued to ring unanswered over several days of trying to reach her. Since I always tried to schedule my calls at a time when she would be in her room, but not so late in the evening that she might be sleeping, I became increasingly concerned that something was amiss.

Eventually, I decided to ring the care home's main number. I spoke to an assistant who said that the reason I was unable to speak with Edith was that she wasn't feeling well. She suggested I leave it for at least a week or two before trying again.

A fortnight later, with Edith's phone remaining unanswered, I rang and spoke to another member of staff who sounded extremely cagey. She told me that Edith was still not well enough to speak to anyone. When I asked her what was wrong with my friend there was an ominous silence. Finally she said, "You'll have to speak to her daughter. I can't say anything else if you're not a member of her family. I'm sorry."

Anxious to find out what was the matter with Edith and when she might be available to take my calls, I contacted her daughter. She informed me that her mother had been suffering from severe back pain and had undergone blood tests to determine the cause. Unable to find any reason for her pain the only other option was to carry out further tests in hospital. Apparently, Edith was not responding well to any tablets for the pain so staff at the care home had said it would be unkind to subject her mother to any invasive tests at this stage in her life and, given the fact that it was believed that mentally she was in decline, Edith's daughter had been asked for her consent to allow a morphine pump to be fitted, which would keep Edith comfortable and pain-free as she would be able to deliver a dose of the medicine whenever she felt she needed it. It would not be possible for me to talk to Edith as she was now terribly confused and heavily sedated from the morphine.

It wasn't my place to protest, to ask whether Edith herself had been consulted about this decision to place her on an end of life pathway. I had no right to cause her daughter further distress, to question whether alternative intervention might have been the kinder option in the long term from Edith's point of view.

Knowing my friend would probably never again be able to converse with me, suspecting that she had never been party to a decision that would precipitate her death, as soon as I replaced the receiver I burst into tears.

Just a couple of weeks earlier Edith had been chatting happily on the phone. I wracked my brain to recall any mention of back pain but there had been none throughout the half an hour we'd spoken.

The following day I rang the care home and spoke to a care worker who, from the manner in which she spoke about Edith, was clearly very fond of her.

"I know that I cannot speak to Edith," I told her "but please will you give her a big hug from me and tell her I love her".

"I'll go in to see her right now," she replied, "and I'll do exactly as you've asked."

It was no surprise when, three weeks later, Edith's daughter phoned me.

"My mother passed away peacefully last night." she said. "At least she wasn't in any pain."

A cold shiver ran down my spine. If Edith had been given a say in the decision about her treatment, might she have possibly chosen a different option from the one that ended her life so precipitately?

Chapter Five

Growing up I was encouraged by my aunt to spend some time visiting the nursing home she ran for elderly folk who were no longer able to live independently. I used to go round there sometimes after school. I particularly remember the delighted expression on the face of one woman whenever I popped my head round her bedroom door. She loved me to sit with her and talk about everything I had learnt at school that day.

And in the room next door to her was a blind lady who would always ask me to describe everything I could see in the garden below, in minute detail. I was her window onto the world, giving her a clear view of the birds, plants and changing seasons. For a time, she said, she was able to 'see' far beyond the limits of her disability.

The home was comfortably furnished, airy and spotlessly clean. My aunt was meticulous in her consideration of the individual needs of every person within its walls. Most importantly, the atmosphere was invariably warm and friendly with plenty of staff around to attend to residents' needs in a calm, unhurried manner.

I actually enjoyed my visits there; I have pleasant memories.

When I was told, in my early fifties, that I needed a operation to correct a prolapsed womb (my only downside of giving birth to five children), I began to make plans for the necessary convalescent period which would follow.

I was fortunate enough to have a husband who was willing to keep an eye on our lively teenage offspring while I took time off from my fulltime job as a Primary School teacher to recuperate.

However, places to convalesce weren't that easy to find and I quickly drew a blank. But it occurred to me that it might be easier to find a nursing home where I could go to rest and recover in peace and quiet.

I did some research and decided I'd rather like to stay in a care home on the coast. I figured that gentle daily strolls in the sea air would hasten my recovery.

I phoned to explain my plan to the manager. Although very amiable, she was somewhat surprised when I explained the reason for my call. All her residents were over sixty-five years old, she told me, many with long-term physical illnesses and disabilities. Nevertheless, for no more than the cost of a week's holiday in a mid- range hotel, she was happy to let one of her ensuite rooms and provide any basic medical care needed.

When I was discharged from hospital the day after surgery, Andrew drove me straight to the home where we were personally warmly welcomed by the manager. Having shown us to my room on the second floor of the old rambling Victorian house, she left me with the promise of a tray with tea for two in a short while.

Though in some need of updating (I think 'tired-looking' might best describe it), it was a reasonable- sized room with a television, soft lighting and a clean adjoining shower and toilet complete with toiletries.

I was relaxing on the comfortable bed when Andrew answered a knock on my door and carried in the promised tea and a plate of biscuits.

Andrew left to make the hour-long journey home, confident that I would be well cared for.

During my time there I saw little of the other residents. At my request, I had all my meals in my room and felt fully rested and refreshed when it was time for Andrew to collect me. I'd passed my days wandering around the large, rambling garden, walking by the sea, reading and watching TV. Any time I required painkillers someone was on hand to promptly dispense them. The staff invariably had a smile and a kind word which, added to the calm atmosphere, ensured that my stay was unexpectedly enjoyable.

Clearly, my positive experience was based on a totally different situation from one where a person is pretty much obliged to remain in the place for the rest of their life. I was relatively young, could come and go as I pleased and was probably considerably more mobile than the other residents. However, I'm sure that the way I was treated reflected the ethos of that home. From the top down, every member of staff I came into contact with conveyed a caring, compassionate attitude by the tone of voice they used whenever they spoke and by prompt attention to my needs. I don't believe for one moment that I had been singled out for special treatment.

In fact, I was so satisfied with this initial recuperate stay that I was ready to repeat it if it were ever again to become necessary (though it would never reach the top of my list of holiday choices).

Chapter Six

When, two years later, I required an operation to wash out my sinuses I didn't anticipate any need for significant recovery time afterwards. I'd already had a similar procedure before and had been well enough to return to teaching within the same week.

However, although the surgery was uneventful, the following morning I had the most horrendous vomiting and diarrhoea imaginable. It's difficult to describe what happened in polite terms but it felt as though my body had suddenly decided to eject everything in it.

Unable to move from the bed, I rang the emergency bell to ask for a bedpan. Unfortunately, before the nurse was able to get it for me, the contents of my stomach and bowels emptied involuntarily onto the sheets.

I kept apologizing whilst two dedicated

nurses screened off my bed and braved the dreadful stench in an attempt to clean me up.

The trouble was that, no sooner had they washed me and changed my bedding than the whole ordeal began again. I began to think it would never end.

I was immediately moved out of the ward into a side room where a doctor quickly set up a drip and injected medication to calm my inflamed insides. Thoroughly weakened and exhausted, I finally drifted off to sleep.

When I woke up, I was puzzled by nurses and doctors nipping in and out to adjust the different tubes and machines I was now linked up to.

I didn't understand what was happening and why. One minute I'd been almost ready to leave the hospital following routine surgery and the next I'd been plunged into the sort of scenario you might expect to see on a TV hospital drama.

It transpired that I was in a single occupancy

room adjoining the cardiac unit. A doctor informed me that the good news was that my heart had not been damaged by the unusual reaction I'd had to Keflex – the antibiotic I'd been given after the operation. But I didn't think, at the time, to question why I was being barrier nursed, why the nurses and doctors always wore masks and aprons to attend to me.

And when my family visited they were obliged to don protective gear. We simply accepted that everyone was doing their best for me, which indeed they were, but the reason for it was not disclosed.

It would be several years before I happened to see my medical records and spotted that my near-fatal state at that time was due to my having contracted clostridium difficile. I had not been allergic to the antibiotic I'd been given, though the Keflex might have left me more vulnerable to contracting this nasty infection of the colon. The hospital had evidently decided to cover up the truth, perhaps concerned about the rising rates of this type of infection in hospital settings. I had, in fact, been lied to.

It took two weeks for me to recover sufficiently to leave the hospital but I was in no way near ready to return to work. I was fatigued and felt terribly weak on discharge. So Andrew decided to arrange for me to spend a week in a nursing home again.

As the place I'd previously stayed at was now full, he booked me into a residence in a nearby country village.

At that point I had scant interest in my surroundings; I simply wanted a quiet, comfortable space where I could spend most of the time sleeping.

However, when I wasn't asleep I couldn't help noticing that the room I'd been allotted was small, rather dark with a small window fairly high up. I figured that I was probably in a basement. Nevertheless, I consoled myself with the fact that I was only here for a short while.

I was treated kindly; my meals were brought to me on a tray and my dirty washing was taken away to be laundered. But I wasn't impressed with the fact that I wasn't asked about whether I wished my name to be written in indelible pen inside my underwear. When I mentioned the labelling issue to the next person to enter my room, she remarked that they had no choice other than to write everyone's name on their clothing in order to ensure that garments were returned to the correct owner once they had been washed and ironed.

I simply didn't have the energy to argue the point that, whilst I understood that there needed to be some system in place to identify residents' clothes, it would have been courteous to at least have my agreement before printing my name on every garment.

A week in that home, whilst providing me with space to recover my strength, left me feeling depressingly like a prisoner confined to a cell with the main difference being that I was not locked in and could have opted to leave at any time.

I have to admit that when Andrew arrived to take me back home I was relieved to leave my dismal surroundings. Once outside, breathing the fresh country air I felt re-invigorated and so glad that I didn't have to remain there a moment longer. At no point had anyone asked whether I might have liked a short break outside in a wheelchair.

Chapter Seven

In 2003, although I was in good shape physically, my mental health began to take a turn for the worse.

The long-standing head of the school, where I had taught fulltime for the previous eight years, retired. She had been an outstanding leader who had gained the respect of everyone who'd worked for her. She had always treated everyone fairly. Children, parents and staff liked and respected her.

Sadly her replacement, although striving to do the best for every child (most of whom came from deprived backgrounds) was far less sensitive to staff's needs. Within a short time a bullying culture developed. A member of staff, who had taught in that school for fifteen years, suffered a complete mental breakdown and didn't return to the classroom. And a newly-qualified teacher, who had begun her teaching career full of enthusiasm, was repeatedly told that the behavioural problems she was experiencing with some children in her class were a result of her poor class management. She frequently came into my classroom in tears at the end of the day. I attempted to reassure her that she had a class with several known behaviourally challenging children who would be difficult for even a more experienced teacher to handle. She really desperately needed support.

Her distress prompted me to go to the head and explain how bad things were for her. I was firmly reminded that I was not her mentor and that I had no right to interfere in anything that didn't concern me, that it was absolutely none of my business.

I had hoped that my intervention might improve the situation for that young teacher. Yet she continued to be told that she, not the children, was the problem; no additional support was put in place for her either in the classroom or for her psychological health. I watched helplessly as her sense of self esteem and self worth plummeted further. I worried also that my own attempts to make the head fully aware of her difficulties and to highlight the fact that she had been given an exceptionally large number of children with complex problems to deal with might actually have made things worse.

All I know is that a week or so later she was off sick with stress and never returned to the classroom.

Moreover, this event triggered deterioration in the head's attitude towards me. She suggested that I take a redundancy that was becoming available, which was not at all what I wanted.

She frequently sat in to observe my lessons which I found particularly nerve-wracking, knowing how she felt towards me. Her explanation was always the same - it was my appraisal. Ofsted descending on our school and singling me out for particular praise for my quality of teaching meant that she no longer had an excuse to constantly sit in on my lessons. But she found various other ways to harass me, loading me with extra responsibilities and showing a distinct lack of sympathy when my mother passed away.

The accumulation of work and personal stress eventually became too much for me. The clinical psychologist I had been seeing for a few months advised me to take a break from teaching but, unwisely, I continued to teach.

I rang the education department and asked if I could be penalised for taking time off for stress. I was informed that it could possibly lead to disciplinary action.

I enjoyed teaching but knew that I was running on empty with few resources to deal with the ongoing tensions at school and increasingly troublesome memories of my past. It didn't help that I was sleep deprived. Every night I would lie awake tortured by flashbacks from my abusive childhood. Eventually I became suicidal.

On my next visit to the psychologist he waited patiently until I finished crying before telling me that I urgently needed to go to the psychiatric department to get admitted. He phoned the hospital to explain to them the gravity of my mental state. I felt I had no choice other than to do as he suggested.

Chapter Eight

I spent several months in the psychiatric ward, dosed up on various medications which were meant to relieve my depression and anxiety and enable me to reach the stage where I could function normally again.

It didn't help that I was in the early phase of the menopause and my hormones were all over the place. Even before my breakdown I had been experiencing the sudden mood swings that so often occur at this stage of life. The bullying - the trigger for my illness - had taken place at a time when I was at my most vulnerable and was totally ill-equipped to deal with it.

Antipressants can work wonders for some people, helping them to regain a footing on normallty sufficiently to move on with their lives. Unfortunately, every tablet or combination of medications that doctors gave me proved disastrous. I was warned that it can take a considerable time to find the most suitable dose of the correct medication for any individual. There is no one size that fits all because people can react differently to any particular drug. In practice, it appears to merely be a case of trial and error (in my case mostly error), until the correct dosage of the most appropriate medication can be found to help someone.

Some of the drugs I was given left me feeling, acting and, probably, looking like a zombie. Others had severe side effects like fainting and stomach pains. Occasionally, a drug appeared to work for a week or so before ceasing to have any positive impact. And then there were the extremely unpleasant withdrawal effects each time a drug was tapered off and another introduced.

It would be another five years before a psychiatrist finally concluded that there wasn't any drug that could help me. Apparently, I just happen to be too sensitive to all the medications designed to treat my condition. By that point I had run the gamut of the entire list!

I did not, of course, stay on an acute psychiatric ward for five years.

My GP had taken me down the path of early retirement on health grounds during my first year's absence from work and I spent much of my time trying to immerse myself in artwork to escape the way I felt. I would spent days at a time in the little summer house in our garden, using oils to depict scenes that transported me temporarily to peaceful, happier places. I painted many fields of vivid red poppies and glowing sunsets. Eventually, I also received therapy which was intended to help me deal with past issues.

Chapter Nine

The waiting list for treatment for dealing with past trauma was lengthy but after two years I finally received an invitation to attend sessions of psychodynamic therapy.

I felt really relieved when I was finally assessed and accepted for this place. At last, I thought I was on the right track to understanding and learning how to deal with my problems. I would have someone to guide me through the maze, help me to cope with life in a positive, constructive manner...

And then I was introduced to Nadia.

Initially things looked hopeful. She asked me about myself and what sort of therapies I'd had before. That took up the first ten minutes of the session. And then she seemed to dry up. She relaxed back into the chair opposite me and said nothing. Of course I waited for more questions, perhaps some direction...

But the silence continued, became difficult, uncomfortable.

The next three sessions were the same; apart from the initial greeting Nadia simply sat and watched me, her face totally impassive.

Nervously, I talked randomly about various childhood incidents, briefly mentioned bullying I'd experienced without being specific. In fact anything that came into my head. But I didn't know yet if I could trust Nadia enough to open up about the severe abuse I'd suffered throughout my childhood.

Occasionally she'd make a comment such as, "Mmm... that seems to leave you feeling frustrated / lonely / sad..."

But I knew that anyway. It was quite obvious even to me, from the way I spoke about things, what my feelings were. I'm not *that* stupid.

During our third session together I began to feel myself getting more and more irritable. I was hoping for some questions, helpful comments that might enable me to know what to speak about. I felt that if she'd asked a few pertinent questions, or even one, it would help me to summon up sufficient courage to talk openly, to feel that she was actually interested in what had happened to me.

"What do you want me to talk about?" I asked her.

Nadia smiled but says nothing.

"It's not funny! I don't know what I'm supposed to be doing. It's not helping me rambling on about this and that," I muttered

"You're angry," she stated calmly. Her expression seemed smug, superior. I felt humiliated.

"Of course I'm angry! I don't need a psychologist to tell me *that*!" I retorted

She didn't respond. How *dare* she sit there, letting me talk round in circles, wind myself up further and further into a frantic frenzy, I thought.

"You get paid for sitting there doing nothing," I accused her. "Just telling me things I already know!"

Still she didn't react; not a flicker of emotion.

I watched the clock, resolved to spend the remaining time in silence, if that's what she wanted. I felt angry and frustrated and passed the next ten minutes studying pictures on the walls. Nadia's eyes remain firmly fixed on my face.

Finally the discomfort became too much. I felt too self-conscious. So I began to waffle about the style of the artist who created the paintings around us. It was all I could think of to talk about.

Nadia simply sat silently watching me.

Suddenly I burst out in exasperation, "What a waste of time this is! And *I* don't even get paid for it." I couldn't think of anything else to say. It was like talking to a robot. If she were really human she'd have seen how lost, how helpless, how hopeless I felt.

I avoided looking at her, tried to pretend she wasn't there. I planned how I'd arrange this room if it were in my house.

"That's it!" Her voice startled me back to reality.

"I'll see you next week," I said lamely.

"No you won't. I'm not seeing you anymore."

The finality of her dismissal hit me like a stone.

"You can't *do* that! I know it's not working but I'm willing to come each week to see if I can get *some*where. You can't give up on me like this." I pleaded.

"It's over," she said firmly, decisively. I could see she wass not going to change her mind

"Well, sod you!" I exclaimed angrily, glaring directly into her eyes.

I turned, walked away fast. For a second I

was tempted to rush back, apologise, plead with her to forgive me, give me another chance. But I knew it would be pointless. She'd clearly written me off.

Chapter Ten

Predictably it would be a considerable wait to access any further help. And as the months lengthened into years my depression deepened. I wasn't getting any better and the changing stream of newly-prescribed antidepressants didn't seem to help, some of them even exacerbating my depression. I wasn't ill enough to be hospitalized but Sarah, my Community Mental health worker, felt that an occasional short spell in a care home might be helpful. It would, in any event, be a change of scene and perhaps motivate me to express myself through my art instead of spending whole days at a time in bed.

So she booked me a week's stay in a large house in a local village where they catered for people of all ages with learning difficulties. I couldn't understand how I fitted into that category but Sarah said that they were willing to take me and that was really all that mattered. Having lost the confidence I'd once had, I was in no position to argue.

On arrival the following afternoon, I was ushered into a small room on the third floor of a large Victorian building, given a time for supper that evening and left to my own devices for the next couple of hours. I sat on the upright chair in one corner of the room and waited, unsure what to do with myself. Every so often I could hear people shouting and doors banging, which frightened me.

At 5.30pm I went downstairs and was directed to a long line in the dining room to await my turn, with all the other residents, for my supper tray. "Hurry up, you're holding up the queue," the woman serving me said brusquely as I stood staring at my plate. I headed for an empty table, next to a window at the far end of the room, hoping that nobody would decide to join me. I felt wary of the other residents who seemed to be rather unpredictable in their behaviour. During the short time I'd been downstairs, one lady uttering obscenities had been practically dragged out by staff, her arms and legs flailing, and an elderly man was stubbornly refusing to eat any of his meal. I'm not sure though that the slice of bread and butter, thinly spread with strawberry jam, the chocolate cupcake and the plastic beaker containing weak tea actually qualified as a 'meal'. None of us had been given any choice. It was simply a question of eating what you were given.

I was relieved that no-one had decided to occupy the two free seats at my table. I didn't mind that most of the residents didn't seem to notice me; a couple of men had stared at me for longer than felt comfortable but otherwise I didn't seem to have attracted any attention, even from the two members of staff who were patrolling the room. Watching them reminded of the movies I'd watched of prison guards on the outlook for any spark of trouble brewing. Perhaps they were oblivious to my presence or had simply accepted any previous notification of my temporary stay and been informed that I didn't require any ongoing monitoring. Whatever the case, a brief check to see if I'd settled in OK, even a smile in my direction would have been welcome; it might even have helped slightly to lift my intense feelings of sadness.

I returned my tray to the counter and returned to my bedroom. Even though it was only shortly after six the late autumn evening had plunged an already dark space into total blackness. I switched on the overhead light and, turned on the television in an attempt to occupy myself, though my concentration waned rapidly with pictures and commentaries on depressing world news events blurring into the background.

At exactly nine o'clock, the allotted time I'd been given for medication when I'd arrived, I went downstairs. A short queue to the dispensing window had already formed along the narrow corridor. By the time I'd taken my sleeping tablet and was on my way back to my room the queue snaked for a few yards around the corner to the stairs. Several of the residents were becoming argumentative with each other which alarmed me; what if one of them decided to pick a fight with me? I hurried past them as fast as I could without actually breaking into a run and possibly causing them to notice me.

I unpacked the few belongings I'd brought with me and washed at the small sink in the corner of my room before getting into bed. Despite the sleepiness induced by the medication, I was painfully aware of the mattress being dreadfully uncomfortable. I tried lying on back, on my side, curled up... but no matter what position I adopted, I could not avoid the mass of lumpy bumps.

Eventually I must have fallen asleep through sheer exhaustion because when I awoke the clock on the wall opposite my bed indicated that it was 8am. When I tried to get up, aware that I was supposed to be at breakfast at eight o'clock, I noticed that the mattress had sagged heavily in the middle making it an effort to get out of the bed. I lifted one side of the mattress to discover that two of the supporting wooden slats were broken. At some point during the night my tossing and turning must have caused the bed to collapse.

When I'd eaten the bowl of cornflakes and the buttered piece of toast - the sole fare on offer - I plucked up courage needed to approach one of the staff to tell them about the broken bed and the unfit- for- use mattress.

"No problem, I'll make a note of it in the book of repairs," she informed me. "With any luck you'll get a replacement today."

The rest of that day passed with no news about either the bed or the mattress. And, because I lacked the mental energy to pursue my complaint, the remainder of my week was spent sleeping with my pillows partially filling the gap created by the damaged bed.

I left that care home as inconspicuously as I'd arrived. I was signed out without anyone enquiring about whether my time there had been satisfactory or not. I derived absolutely no benefit from being there.

I'm sure that a new bed would have had to be found for the next temporary or permanent resident but I'm not so convinced that they wouldn't have inherited that same mattress.

Chapter Eleven

I did briefly mention the bed to Sarah yet perhaps she'd forgotten about it when, several months later, she phoned to tell me she'd reserved a place for me in a different facility. I'd struggled on but recently hadn't felt motivated to do any artwork or indeed anything else and Sarah felt that, even though there was no need to for me to be hospitalized, being somewhere different might inspire me to paint again.

"This home should really suit you," she stated, "It's practically on the beach and I remember you said that you used to love holidays by the sea."

I was sorely tempted to turn down the offer of what Sarah now termed 'respite' but she'd told me that she had gone to great lengths to procure this spot, that I was lucky to get it. So, not wanting to appear ungrateful for her efforts, I reluctantly accepted and put my brushes, paper and tubes of paint in my suitcase to take with me.

Sarah was right in that the care home was indeed a mere two minute walk from the promenade, which overlooked a seemingly never-ending stretch of golden sand. I hoped that a combination of warmer weather and sea breezes would improve my mood. And, when I arrived I felt a little encouraged by the care assistant who had a welcoming smile on her face as we made our way up the stairs to the third floor of this four storey building.

She opened the door to a bedroom which, although perfectly fitting the descriptive word 'tired' used by estate agents to avoid describing any property as in need of a drastic overhaul, was spacious and airy.

There was no ensuite but the still smiling assistant took me to a bathroom a couple of doors to the right of my room, which I took to be for my use. I was unclear whether other residents also had access to it but had to assume that they probably did since it was evident, from her response to my question, that this lady spoke very little English. "Teatime downstairs, six o'clock," she said pointing to her wristwatch, to make sure I understood.

With ample time until then, I laid down on my bed to rest, relieved to find that the mattress was firm and comfortable. Exhausted after the two hour car journey, I soon dozed off and the next thing I knew it was five minutes to six.

It became clear on entering the massive dining room that this place was home to adults of all ages who were mentally challenged. Mostly, however, they seemed calmer than the previous home I'd stayed in. A few of them greeted me briefly and a number of others smiled at me.

My hopes of sitting on my own faded as a middle aged lady ambled over to the corner table where I was sitting, sat down without a word and proceeded to tuck noisily into her baked potato and salad. Although we were given no choice about what food was served up, it was, nevertheless, plentiful and well-cooked.

The next couple of days passed fairly uneventfully. I'd finally got round to unpacking my art equipment and hoped to get started on a picture soon; I'd even ventured out for a walk each day. Taking off my sandals and focusing on the warm sand as I strolled along the beautiful stretch of beach, certainly seemed to have lifted my spirits a little. Maybe Sarah was right, perhaps this break would turn things around for me and I would be able to get my life back on track. Then I would at long last be able to enjoy being retired.

Returning from an early evening walk I happened to glance up at the roof of the care home with its tall round tower silhouetted against a glorious sunset. I wondered if anyone ever went up into that part. Perhaps it wasn't even accessible now.

Once inside the building, I mounted the stairs

to my bedroom but paused when I noticed a small door diagonally to my right. There was no-one around up here and judging by its position that door might possibly lead to that tower, I reckoned. I crossed the landing and turned the door handle; the heavy wooden door opened easily. Ahead of me a loomed a steep, narrow staircase. I listened for a moment to make sure I was alone then, unable to resist the temptation to explore, I closed the door quietly behind me and started to climb the worn steps. The staircase curved slightly before opening onto what was obviously the inside of the tower with sash windows on all sides. I was astonished and somewhat taken aback to see that one of the sash windows was partially open. There must be inevitably be a restrainer on it preventing it from opening more than the few inches It currently was, I reasoned. To check, I pulled at the window using both hands. To my horror it slid all the way up, leaving a sufficiently large gap for anyone to actually fall out if they were to lean out. I gasped and heaved the window down until it slammed safely shut.

What if one of the residents were to find their way up here? That open window could prove lethal. I shuddered at the thought as I made my way back to the comparative safety of my bedroom, making sure that I had firmly closed the door to the tower.

Andrew dropped in on me for a surprise visit shortly after supper. "What's up?" he said as soon as we were seated in the small room reserved for visitors. "I could see straight away, from the expression on your face, that something is bothering you."

"I'm really worried," I confided. I related the entire incident to him, finally expressing my concern for the other residents, given their sometimes unpredictable and extreme behaviours. " I don't want to complain," I told him, " but that unlocked door is a danger."

Assuring me that he would handle the matter

as tactfully as possible, Andrew went off in search of the manager. He was back after a few minutes. "OK, luckily the manageress is on duty and I've had a word. She is going to lock that door and warn all staff about keeping it locked."

I thanked him for dealing with the matter and just hoped that there would be no further recurrence.

I'd forgotten about the incident by the following afternoon when I was stopped in the corridor by a tall, thin woman who introduced herself as the person in charge of the care home.

"I understand that you went up to the tower yesterday," she said brusquely. "You had no business being up there, it's for staff only."

"But the door wasn't locked," I protested. "Well it is now," she said decisively," before turning on her heel and disappearing into the office.

I felt bruised by her attitude; she'd made it

sound as if somehow I was the one who was at fault.

That night I set my alarm as usual to wake me in good time to get ready for breakfast. But the next morning when I reached out my right arm to turn it off, I misjudged the distance between my bed and the bedside table and fell sideways into the gap between them. As I landed heavily onto my right side, I heard a sudden crack and felt a sharp pain shoot through my body. I tried to get up but the pain was so great that I was unable to move.

I don't know how long I lay there moaning, unable to even get to my phone to get help. Eventually, I must have been missed when I didn't show up for breakfast because the bedroom door opened and a voice called out to me to hurry up if I still wanted something to eat as they were starting to clear away the dishes.

I shouted that I was on the floor and had hurt myself badly. I was just wondering how much longer I would have to lie helplessly on the cold hard floor when I heard footsteps heading towards me.

"Right, there are two of us so we'll get you up now." I recognized the clipped, efficient tone of the manageress. "You take her that side," she directed her assistant.

I screamed out in agony as someone attempted to lift my right arm.

"Stop that at once!" the manageress demanded, "You'll disturb the other residents. "There's absolutely no need to make all this fuss."

"I'm sorry," I sobbed, "but I really need to go to hospital. I'm sure I've broken something. It hurt so much when you tried to move me. Please ring for an ambulance."

She let out a long sigh. "OK, have it your way. But this is totally unnecessary. You've probably just bruised yourself. You're not even trying to help yourself."

Undoubtedly feeling she had no other option, she dialed the emergency services as I'd asked before turning on her heel and walking out. The assistant who'd accompanied her remained and, as soon as the door was closed, sat down beside me. "Don't mind her," she said kindly. "She's like that with most people, especially if they get on the wrong side of her. And she was ranting at hand-over this morning about the fact that you'd made a complaint about the tower door even though you were right to mention it because it should always have been kept locked. In fact I'm surprised that there hasn't been an accident before now."

It was probably only a few minutes, but felt like an eternity, before the door opened and I heard someone say, "She's on the floor the other side of the bed."

A wave of relief flooded through me on hearing the gentle, tone of the paramedic who was examining me. "I can see that your collarbone took the full impact of your fall.

You've almost certainly fractured it, but don't worry we'll get it sorted," he reassured me.

Having ascertained that I did not lose consciousness and that I didn't have any pain apart from my shoulder, he carefully put my arm into a sling and, together with his co-worker, helped me downstairs and into the waiting ambulance. As soon as I was seated on the stretcher, he said he was going to give me something for the pain. He put a mask over my mouth and instructed me to breathe deeply and evenly.

As the gas and air began to take effect, I floated thankfully into a totally pain-free zone for the remainder of the journey to hospital.

Unfortunately for me, once we arrived at A&E I had to be disconnected from the machine and the pain crept back.

An x-ray revealed the broken collar bone, which could only be treated by keeping that arm in a sling for six weeks, the doctor told me. He stressed that I must keep it very still at all times and discharged me with a prescription for strong morphine-based painkillers.

As soon as I'd finished my consultation with the doctor, a woman approached me and introduced herself.

"I'm Marion, the cook at the care home. I followed the ambulance to hospital. I was the only one available after your accident to make sure you had return transport."

As we made our way to her car, she told me that she would stop off on the journey back to get my script filled. She emerged from the pharmacy carrying my pain pills and a bottle of water so that I could take a couple immediately. I was grateful for her thoughtfulness, which did not end there because, on our arrival back, the moment she'd switched off the engine she turned to me, checked how I was feeling and said that if there was anything at all I needed, I only had to ask.

I thanked her and headed slowly and painfully up the stairs to my bedroom. Despite the fact that it was my collar bone that was damaged, the rest of my body felt bruised and ached dreadfully. When I finally reached my room, I lay down on my bed. The medication had made me drowsy and all I wanted to do was sleep.

It was already dark when I awoke. The house was silent. Had anyone come to check on me whilst I slept, I wondered. The pain in my shoulder felt unbearable. It was barely four hours since I'd taken the painkillers but, unable to stand the blinding agony any longer, I took another dose and spent the rest of the evening and that night dozing fitfully.

It was nine o'clock the following morning when I was suddenly woken by the manageress towering over my bed. "It's high time you got up, "she said briskly. "You've already missed breakfast so just make sure you get down for lunch. You can walk, you haven't broken your leg." With those final words she turned on her heel and walked out of my room closing the door behind her.

Still in immense pain, I was hurt by the fact that she hadn't even asked how I was feeling. Surely she must have noticed that I hadn't even changed into my nightwear last night.

I got up slowly but my head began to swim. I sat down on the bed and sat trying to work out how on earth I was even going to get washed and changed, let alone make it downstairs for lunch later.

By the time my clock reached eleven, I was so frustrated and unhappy at constantly trying and failing to do anything for myself that I was sitting on my bed crying when there was a knock on my door and Marion popped her head round, an anxious expression on her face.

Seeing my distress she came over and sat on my bed.

"Hasn't anyone been in to help you?" she

inquired kindly. I told her what had happened with the manageress and how isolated and helpless I felt.

She frowned but didn't comment except to say, "Well I'm here now to make things easier, you can definitely count on me. I'm just going to get a bowl of water to wash you and then I'll help you get into some clean clothes."

I felt so grateful for Marion's compassionate understanding. She realized that I simply couldn't carry on as normal, doing the ordinary mundane things we all take for granted until we are no longer able to do without help. She was the only person who made the remainder of my stay in that care home bearable. Despite the fact that she must inevitably have been incredibly busy preparing and cooking meals for the other residents, she never once complained about her regular trips to my room with drinks, meals and to help me with getting dressed and undressed. Seeing her friendly face and hearing her soft Welsh accent at frequent intervals throughout the day was also a distraction from the immense pain I was still experiencing.

The day before my discharge Andrew turned up with our eldest son, Mark, who decided that I needed to venture out with them in the wheelchair that they'd managed to borrow from a small collection of them in the basement.

They helped me downstairs. "This wheelchair isn't exactly state of the art," my son exclaimed, as he manoeuvred the chair down the stone steps onto the gravel path and applied the brakes, or at least, tried to. "These brakes are knackered and the tyres are almost flat but it was the least worst out of the ones we were shown. I've dusted it down with a tissue so it'll do."

Holding my son's arm, I cautiously lowered myself onto the seat. The wheelchair was uncomfortable but, nevertheless, I welcomed the experience of being outside, finally breathing in lungfuls of clean, fresh air. I'd almost forgotten how good it felt.

We were out for an hour, with my son struggling to keep the wheelchair moving in the same direction along the promenade. It was quite funny being in something that resembled one of those supermarket trolleys whose wheels don't seem to be designed to work together making it zigzag wildly from one side of the aisle to the other in spite of every attempt to straighten it; but it was also a bit scary as I couldn't be sure I'd arrive back at the home without being accidentally tipped out.

Following my precarious outing, and with Andrew's reassurance that he'd be back early the next afternoon to collect me, I was trying to focus on a magazine I was looking at when Marion came in carrying my supper tray. As she was on the verge of going off duty and wouldn't be in the following day, she said she would sit with me for a short while. She'd left strict written instructions, she told me, for the assistant cook to make sure I got breakfast and lunch on time.

As we chatted I began to sense her dissatisfaction with the place.

"I shouldn't be saying this, but I'm really angry at the way you've been treated while you've been here. You deserve better." She said in a low voice. The door was closed but she glanced towards it as though afraid of being overheard. "This isn't the first time either. But it's no use making a complaint. Management just isn't interested," she said, with a sigh.

Chapter Twelve

I'd made up my mind that, after my last experience, I was never again going to stay in any care home. However, a year later, shortly before my trauma therapy was due to begin, my mental health was beginning to spiral downhill. Sarah approached me cautiously, knowing the details of what had happened previously.

"I know that you are determined not to have any respite care, " she said, "but you need to be in top shape for this new treatment that you've waited so long to access. This particular home that I have in mind, that I've already been in contact with, is a completely different kettle of fish. I've spoken with Julia, who manages the home and she was absolutely horrified when I relayed what had occurred in the last place you were in. She assures me that the home she works in gives personal attention to each of its thirty residents, many of whom have dementia.

"She wants you to know that your time there would be very different and she's perfectly happy to visit you to discuss any special requirements you may have beforehand. In fact, I've taken the liberty of provisionally arranging for her to come and see you."

Reluctantly, I agreed to meeting up with the manageress the next day. Sarah had gone to a lot of trouble on my behalf and it would be rather churlish of me to refuse the meeting.

And when Julia arrived she was indeed the warm, friendly woman I'd been led to expect. It seemed nothing would be too much trouble. She had a large room with windows facing onto their beautiful country garden, an ensuite, and it was only on the first floor of a two storey house. She presented me with a colourful, brochure, which certainly inspired confidence. If I were to have any problems whatsoever, she told me, I could go to her and she would sort them out straight away. In fact, she went so far as to give me her mobile number so that I would have the facility to do this, in the unlikely event that the need arose.

After an hour in Julia's company, I was sure that she was a woman of her word. So, before she left, she'd arranged for me to come at the beginning of the following week. She would then be able to personally show me around, she said, as she would be on duty then.

The large Edwardian building, set in extensive grounds on the outskirts of a quaint village, looked promising. Julia opened the door looking delighted to see me. She invited me into the wide hallway and accompanied me on a tour of the house beginning with the huge lounge where chairs filled with residents lined the walls. It felt incredibly sad but perhaps the feeling was mine as I surveyed so many expressionless faces.

Julia pointed to a piano at one end of the room. "I've heard that you're quite an accomplished pianist, "she said enthusiastically. "We'd love to hear you play whenever you feel like it. Unfortunately, none of the staff plays and the residents all have dementia so they can't play but they do like listening to music from time to time." I wondered whether the idea had even been suggested to any of the residents. At varying stages of cognitive decline, it was surely possible that one or two of them might still be able to play something, if encouraged. Simply to assume that not a single one of them could possibly be capable of performing seemed rash to me. But, not wishing to appear confrontational in any way, I kept my thoughts to myself.

The room assigned to me was L-shaped. There was ample room to move around and, although the area where the bed was situated was rather dark and narrow, it opened out onto a roomy rectangle. Here the sun shone brightly through wide bay windows which overlooked a large expanse of lawn surrounded by trees and flowering shrubs.

"I think you'll be comfortable here," Julia said. "I'll send up a tray with your lunch and just let me know if there's anything else you need."

I thanked her and unpacked my art materials ready to begin painting that afternoon.

The first couple of days were uneventful and I slowly began to unwind, started to feel a bit more positive. Perhaps Sarah was right and this was the ideal precursor to put me in a better frame of mind for therapy.

Medication was brought to each resident by the night staff at nine o'clock each evening. The staff member then waited until the pills were taken before leaving the room. However, on the third night I was about to pop the prescribed sleeping tablets into my mouth when I noticed that they were a different colour and shape from usual.

When I mentioned this, the nurse shrugged, "Probably a different manufacturer, " she ventured.

Not reassured by her response I asked if she would mind checking the packet or bottle they'd been taken from. Heaving a sigh, she left my room to do as requested. Five minutes later she returned with the oval, white tablets I was familiar with.

She showed me the packet with my name on the front, saying they must have got mixed up with someone else's. It was hardly an apology for what I felt was a serious mistake.

The error with my tablets could have affected another resident who would have mistakenly been given my sleeping medication. They could have missed out on their essential daily dosage for some health condition. And whatever I could have ingested might well have harmed me.

Julia was not on duty that night but, remembering her insistence that I contact her immediately if I was unhappy about anything in the home, I rang her mobile.

She listened quietly until I'd finished telling

her about what had just happened before agreeing that this was negligence that should never have happened since any medication dispensed to a resident was supposed to be checked by another member of staff as a safety measure.

After apologizing profusely, Julia assured me that, although she was not due in the following day she would, nevertheless, arrive for hand-over first thing in the morning to address this issue with the nurse concerned and impress upon her the gravity of the situation.

The next morning I woke feeling ill. Julia popped in to see me to reassure me that she had dealt with the medication mix-up and was sure it was a one off occurrence. She took my temperature and urged me to rest in bed for the day as I'd obviously picked up some bug. She brought me a clean glass, a jug of water and paracetamol for my headache and urged me to drink plenty throughout the day.

I thanked her for her kindness and did as she'd instructed. The only problem was that by lunchtime the jug was empty. I told the care assistant who delivered my lunch tray that I felt too sick to eat anything but asked if she would refill my jug.

She must have forgotten since no-one appeared in my room before the appointed nighttime distribution of medication as far as I could see. In any case my jug didn't reappear.

I dozed on and off but saw nobody; the hours dragged and I felt poorly, rather sorry for myself and wished so much that someone would at least come in to see if I needed anything. Of course they must have been busy with other residents but a brief check on me from time to time wouldn't have taken long and would have meant a lot.

Since meds were regularly distributed at nine o'clock, I knew that someone would turn up at the appointed hour. With still half an hour to go, I was sweating but shivery, my night clothes and the sheet under me were damp. I hated the sensation of them sticking to the plastic surface of the mattress.

A nurse I'd never seen before entered my room and hurriedly handed me my pills without so much as an inquiry as to how I was feeling. She seemed flustered as she headed for the door, clearly intent on moving quickly onto the next resident.

"Hang on a minute," I called out.

Her hand already on the door handle, she turned round. "What is it?" she demanded, a look of impatience on her face.

"You've given me the wrong medication."

"No I haven't, "she retorted, "Those are the ones prescribed for you." Without waiting for a response, she left the room closing the door firmly behind her.

I stared at the two round, brown pills in my hand. How on earth could a mistake of this nature occur again? And how come she didn't even follow protocol, I wondered, and wait until I'd taken them?

I was feeling ill already without making myself even more unwell.

I picked up my phone and rang Julia who was appalled to learn that not only had I not been kept adequately hydrated but had been given what she suspected were Amitriptyline Hydrochloride, which she knew had been prescribed for the patient in the room next to mine.

Unable to bear how badly I felt mistreated, I told Julia that I was going to ring my husband to come and collect me. She urged me to stay, at least until morning as it was now nine thirty, but I insisted that I could not spend a moment longer in the home. I had come here to build up my strength and had ended up feeling so much worse.

Andrew was horrified to hear what had occurred and readily agreed to collect me that night, promising that he would be there within the hour.

Despite feeling weak and dizzy, I began to pack away my art materials and the few belongings I'd brought with me. There was a knock on my door and two staff, a man and a woman, entered the room. Both looked extremely concerned as they approached me.

"We've just had a call from Julia to explain why you are leaving here tonight. We are so sorry. This should never have happened to you. We are really shocked. We are trained nurses," she continued, "but because we come from the Philippines we have to do further training before we are allowed to practice in your country. Here we are only allowed to be care assistants."

It transpired that they were living in accommodation belonging to the owner of the care home who deducted a large proportion of their meager salary for board and lodging, leaving them with little to live on.

"We are very worried about this place," the male nurse told me. "What has happened to you is not the first time with people who stay here. This would not happen in our country. The training for nurses is excellent."

We chatted for a while longer. They were so kind and friendly and I wished I had met them before. At one point they showed me some photos of beautiful scenery in their native country.

Our conversation was abruptly interrupted by a cross face peering round the door.

"There you are!" the nurse who'd issued the wrong medication said in an exasperated tone. "I've been searching everywhere for you. Get on with what you are supposed to be doing right now," she commanded.

Casting me a crestfallen glance, the two assistants left quickly. In spite of their expertise it was clear that they were utterly powerless to change the system. Even attempting to do so would mean losing their jobs.

I was so relieved when Andrew arrived. We left hurriedly, both vowing that this really was the final stay in any care home. My trust had been betrayed too severely.

Chapter Thirteen

In relation to the two staff who came into my bedroom shortly before I left the last care home, insufficient attention is paid to those numerous care staff who are not accorded the appropriate and deserved status or respect by their employers. And yet they form an enormous proportion of the staffing of these places. They are all too frequently overworked and grossly underpaid.

To quote from Mitchell and Strain, (2015):-

"Despite the importance of the care home within UK and international healthcare systems, there has not always been a recognition that care home nurses, and indeed care home care support staff, are specialist practitioners."

I know from speaking with the those two staff from the Philippines' that they were keen to receive any further necessary training but not only had they found it difficult to access further specialist training from the NHS, when they had finally managed to do this they were then expected to attend training sessions in their own very limited free time. They were told that there were not sufficient staff to replace them during their working hours so it was up to them to fit in the extra training whenever they could.

Is it any wonder then that there continues to be a significant problem with recruiting and retaining qualified and competent staff?

Undeniably, continuity of care is paramount when it comes to looking after residents in care homes. And it takes a good while to build trust with an individual, to understand their personal needs and their clinical background.

A high staff turnover remains a difficulty in many homes. To deal with this, agency staff are frequently brought in to fill the gaps but this is clearly unsettling for residents and does not solve the long term, long-standing problems with staffing.

Care homes are an important aspect of any health system. Thanks to advancements in medicine people are increasingly living much longer. The downside of this is that the requirement to provide care for older people with complex needs has expanded rapidly yet, since care homes were privatised, their functioning continues to be somewhat overlooked and neglected by governments. Unfortunately, there is now an inherent danger of profit being the primary driving factor in the private sector.

The Care Quality Commission (CQC) originates from 2009. It was specifically set up to monitor the care given to residents of care homes, amongst other medical establishments, and set targets, where necessary, for improvement.

The last place I was in was inspected twice in 2017 A great number of essential improvements were deemed necessary. The home had a further inspection in 2018 when it was found that the targets set had failed to be met. The following is quoted from the summary of their report:-

"There was not always enough staff on duty with the right skill mix to keep people safe and respond to their care needs in a timely manner. People were at risk of harm from poor infection control practices, environmental issues and poor management of risk factors. Medicines management was not always practiced safely.

"Care staff often worked on their own initiative without supervision and visible leadership. People were not always provided with their choice of food or with a balanced and nutritious diet.

"People and their relatives were not involved in planning their care. Care was not person centered, but was task orientated. Staff had little insight into the needs of people with cognitive problems and poor spatial awareness. There was a high staff turnover and people did not always know the staff looking after them.

"People did not always receive personalised care that was responsive to their needs. Staff did not acknowledge their likes and dislikes."

The home was found to be inadequate and put into special measures. Several months later it closed down permanently. Throughout the years it had been accepting people with a multitude of varying individual needs, it had shown scant regard for them as human beings requiring high quality care. The pain and suffering of those who lived there and of their relatives and friends is unimaginable!

I have read other reports, not merely of places that I spent time in, but also of others where care has been found to be unacceptable and a vast number of significant improvements have been required. Of course, there are, as I've previously mentioned, care homes where each person is looked after with the compassionate care and respect that every single one of us has a right to. Yet, while even one place exists where failure to preserve the dignity and humanity is prevalent, we cannot rest easy. It's high time that we call out any home where indignities, neglect or abuse are prevalent.

Regrettably, my own experiences of time spent in care homes are far from isolated incidences; yet rarely do they hit the headlines in national news. And when they do they are quickly superseded by other news items.

I always had the option to leave, somewhere else to go. But what about the many who are subjected to similar or far worse treatment in such places and don't have any alternative place of residence? It is for every single one of them - the silent sufferers - that I speak out today.

Printed in Great Britain
by Amazon